Lilly's Garden

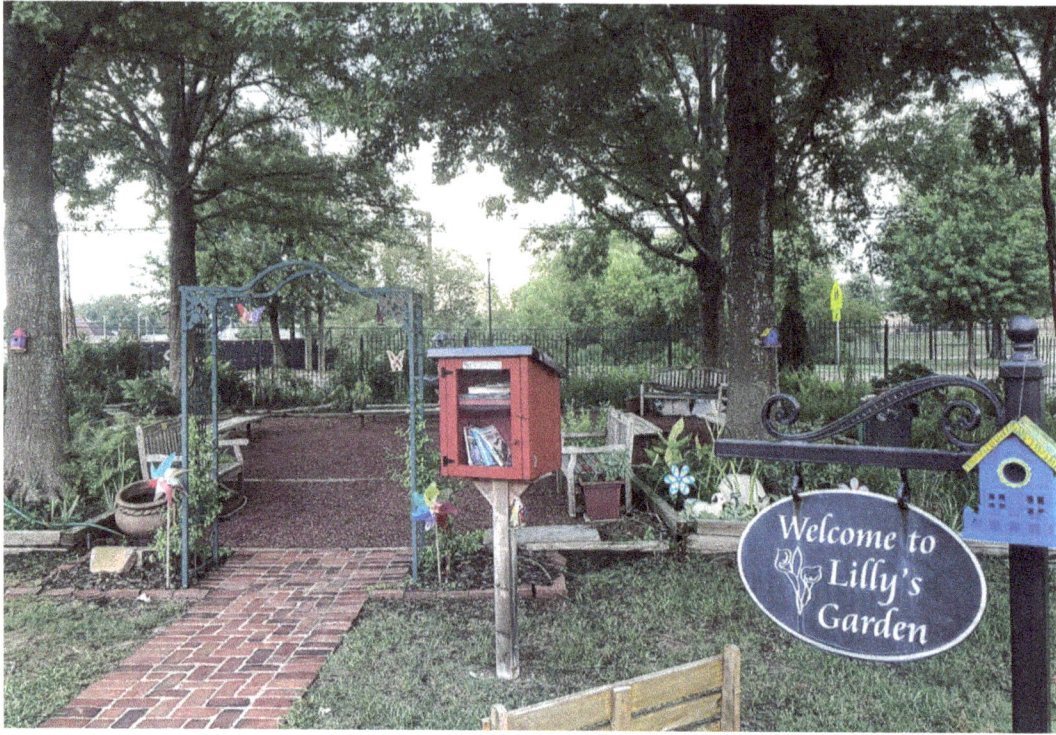

On the grounds of Forest Avenue Magnet Elementary School.

Lilly's Garden

The Story of Lilly, Her Family, and Her Special Legacy

Ann N. Oldham

Black Belt Press

Montgomery

Black Belt Press
105 S. Court Street
Montgomery, AL 36104

Cataloging-in-Publication Data

ISBN-13: 978-1-961938-23-6 (hardback)

Design and composition by Randall Williams

Printed in the United States of America

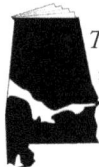

BLACK BELT PRESS | MONTGOMERY

*The Black Belt, defined by its dark, rich soil, stretches across central Alabama. It
was the heart of the cotton belt. It was and is a place of great beauty, of extreme
wealth and grinding poverty, of pain and joy. Here we take our stand, listening to
the past, looking to the future.*

To my loving sons, Jason and Jaylan Thompson, who gave me hope and love at a time when I felt there was little reason to look forward.

To my dear sister, Claire Flennoy, who has loved me and stood by me throughout my life in so many ways.

To my loving husband, Myron H. Thompson, who greets me daily with a bright smile when he walks through the door. Whatever the circumstances, his smile says to me, "Whatever it is, together we can make it work." He has always been my biggest champion.

And in loving memory of Lilly's biggest fan and her best friend, my dear son, Miles Thompson, whom we also lost too soon.

~

Proceeds from this book will help fund the sickle cell disease project — The Lilly and Miles Foundation — and the Lilly Thompson Garden and Outdoor Classroom through the Birmingham Community Foundation.

Lilly Thompson at Forest Avenue Elementary School

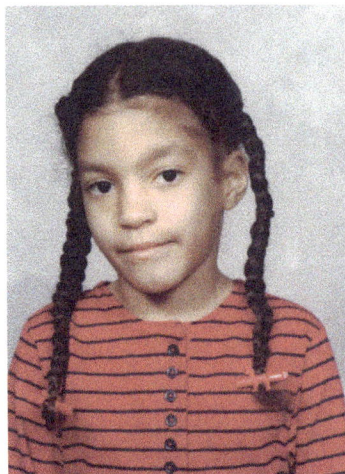

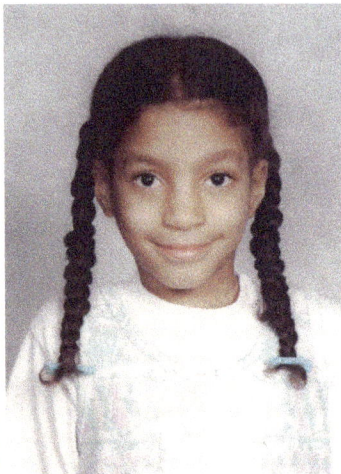

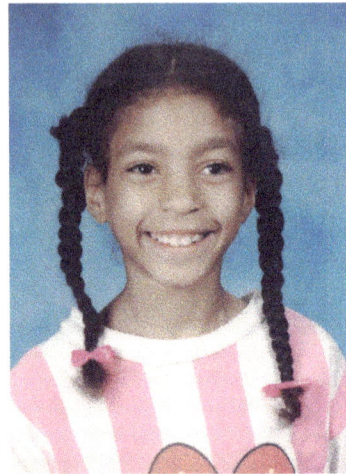

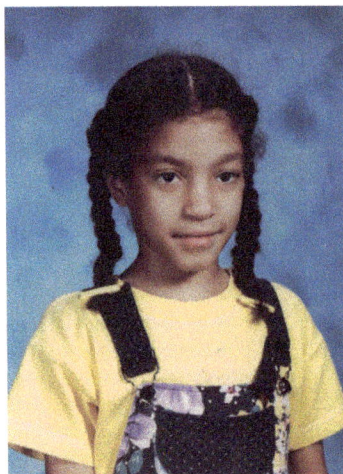

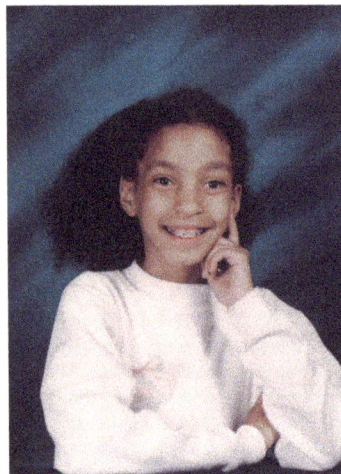

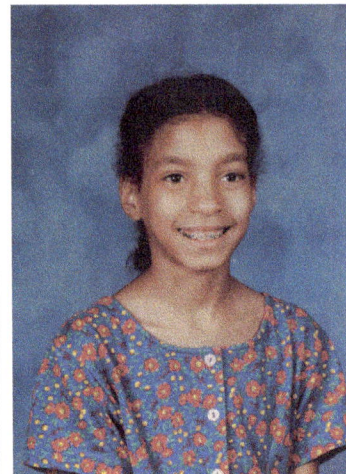

Top row, from left: kindergarten, first grade, second. Bottom: third, fourth, and fifth.

Contents

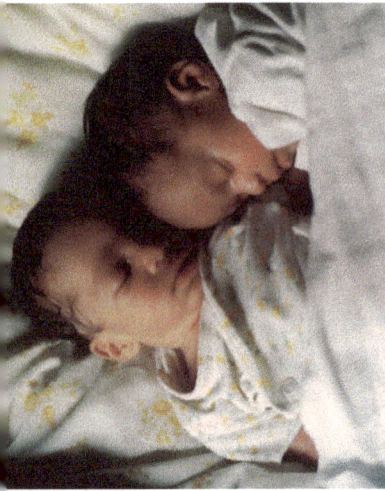

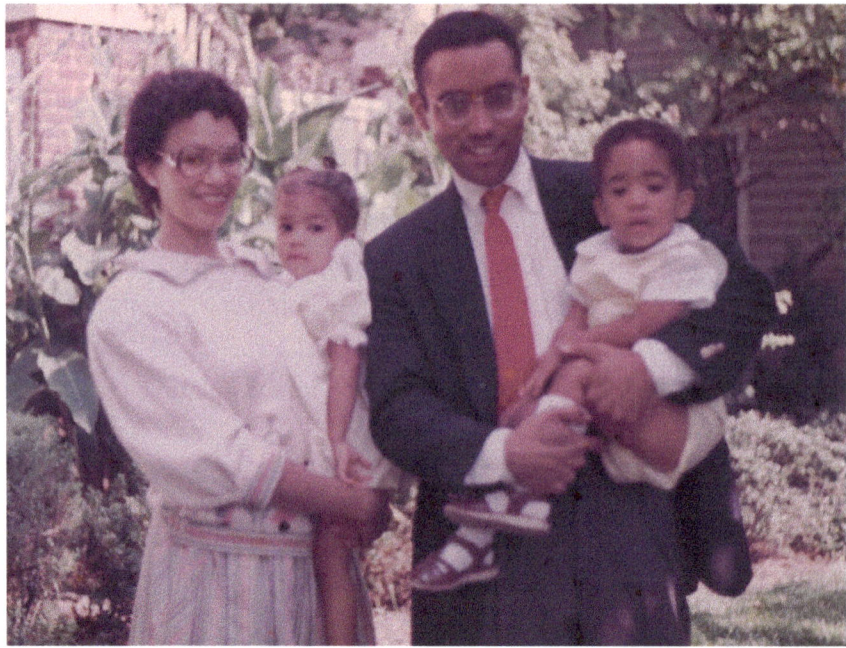

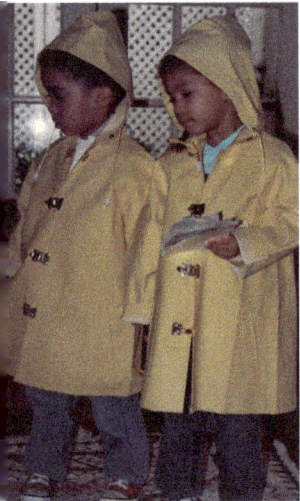

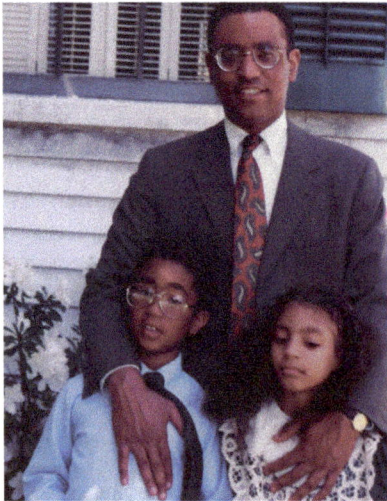

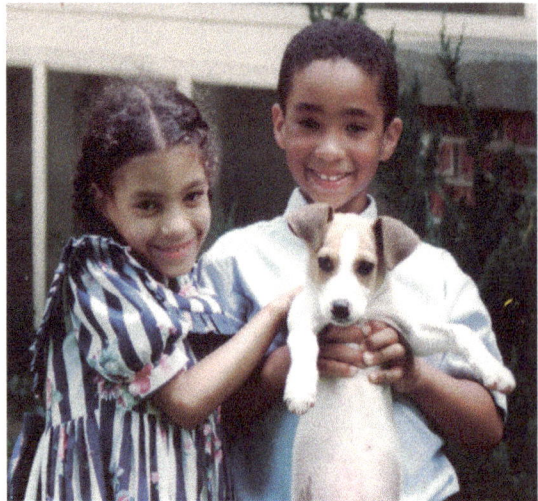

Moments with our twins, Lilly and Miles: Top, one month old, and a year old, Easter 1987. Bottom, from left, three years old; six years old, with Myron; with puppy Max, a gift for their seventh birthday.

Introduction

After losing our precious daughter, Lilly, I tried to fill the void that her absence left in me and in my family. Many days I spent rambling in our old house looking at her things, smelling her clothes to feel her presence. Nothing could replace her.

Dinner time was difficult. Setting the table made her absence even more pronounced. Often we ate with plates in our laps in front of the TV—something I was previously dead set against. Sometime later we moved to the table, but I kept Lilly's place crowded with large plants so it appeared there was no room for another place setting.

I continued to work most days to escape the emptiness I felt at home. But trouble arose when clients came in. I withdrew to the back of the office where I could not be seen by the people I knew.

Time moved on though I was standing still. Our son, Miles, who was ten years old at the time, attended school and resumed his regular activities. After school he shot hoops on our backyard basketball goal. He urged me to watch, and later, to play. I did a little—but it was all I could do not to cry in his presence. He tried hard to pull me along to join him in getting outside of myself. Miles was the kind of person, much like his dad, who greets everyone with a smile—mostly in good spirits unless something is wrong.

That year, Andy Cohen, one of Myron's clerks, made time in her schedule to be with Miles. She taught him to play tennis after

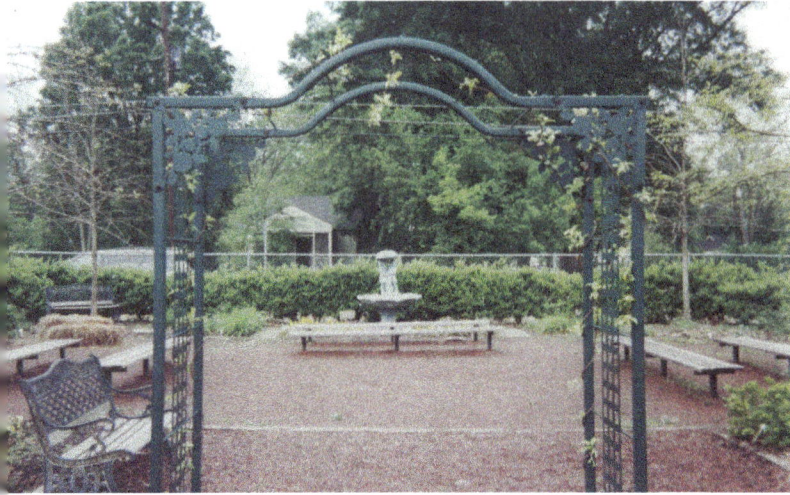

The beginning of Lilly's Garden, 1997.

school and during the summer months. Andy gently urged Miles to try something new and then improve his skills. It saved him from being inactive because of my lack of energy and engagement at that time to encourage him.

During Lilly's memorial service at her school, the original "Save the Earth Club" members announced that the proceeds from the school's recycling campaign would be set aside for the construction of a garden in her name. The "Lilly Pad" is a gift that the fifth grade left to the school. A dedication ceremony was held on May 16, 1997.

Lori Siegelman was instrumental in obtaining state grant funds for a school garden with the principal's specification that it be designed as an outdoor classroom. Because of her advocacy in adopting the garden as a community service project (2001) the Capital City Master Gardeners have not only worked to maintain the beauty of Lilly's Garden, they have sponsored and conducted many programs for every grade level at the school. With the collaboration between the school counselor, Mrs. Shirley Johnson, and the teachers, the Master Gardeners have held programs involving seed science and plant life; Alabama birds and their habitats; the history of telling time and setting a sundial; the study of bees and their importance to our food chain. They have been introduced to composting with food scraps and other household recyclables; the students have made their own science journals; they learned about the famous Alabama scientist, Dr. George Washington Carver; they have planted and harvested sweet potatoes which they donated to a local food pantry. Various classes have done art projects in the garden such as watercolors; painting gourds used as bird houses. Each class made stepping stones that are permanent fixtures in the garden. Many former students return to the garden to find their stepping stone. Activities there can be incorporated in every facet of the school curriculum.

Lilly's Garden sits on a peninsula to the left of the school campus. Some warm summer days passersby enjoy the peaceful shelter of its tall oaks and crape myrtles. Others stop to compliment the master gardener volunteers seen working there. In May, Lilly's birth month, one might catch a glimpse of the beautiful "Lilly's Smile," a special daylily hybridized by Paul Furr of the Daylily Society.

In 2013, Lilly's Garden and Outdoor

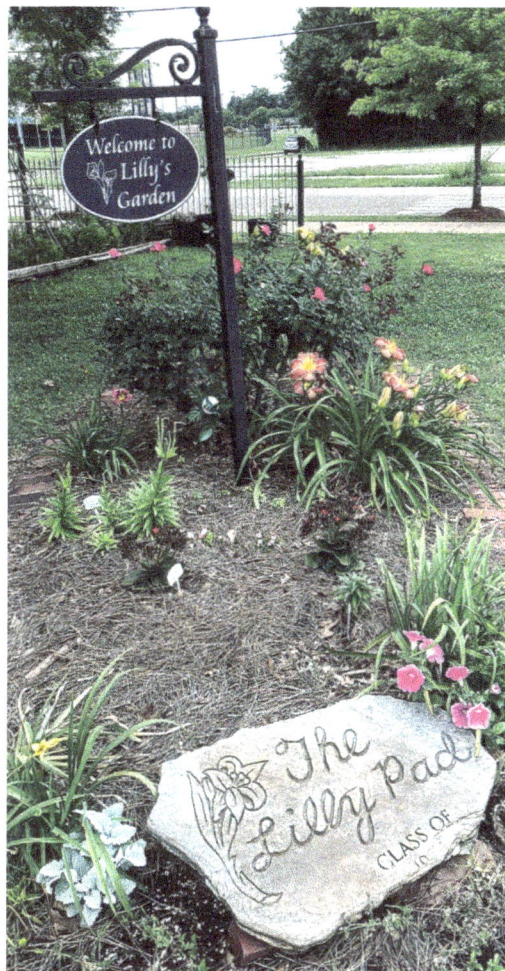

The sixth grade of 1997 left the Lilly Pad as a gift to the school.

Classroom won the state award for gardens in Alabama that teach, beautify, and enhance the community. This award was given by the Alabama Master Gardeners Association.

Lilly's Garden and Outdoor Classroom is a place for learning while maintaining its natural beauty. Our family cannot think of a more fitting memory for our daughter.

No matter what anyone told me, time does help heal. After announcing to my employer that I was going to enroll in a teaching program, I quit my travel agency job and enrolled in a local college. I was interested in special education and reading. I enrolled in two courses to see if I would like teaching. I also enrolled in a writing course to get more practice writing papers for my classes. I liked the writing classes best and was encouraged to improve my skills. I began to write short stories about my children—Lilly and Miles—little incidents that reminded me of the times we had together, small vignettes that revealed their personalities and their relationship to one another. I thought that one day Miles might enjoy telling his children about his sister. I did not want time to steal his memory of her.

While gathering material for the stories, I sometimes asked Miles how he remembered particular incidents. A few of the stories I read to him. The memories involving both children soothed me, and I felt that their connection was so close it could not be undone by the absence of one. In short, Miles would not forget his sister. That was what I wanted.

Haunted House

Halloween night evokes more surprises than one might expect. The Halloween of 1990 was one of the memorable times.

Inside the house a young witch and her companion, a small pirate, donned their costumes, preparing to join their fellow creatures of the night. With a slight bend in the hat and a cocking of the eye patch, the two dashed out into the cold crisp air to meet their companions for a night of looting.

The night sky showed no light except that from the flickering flashlights held by those who scampered along the edges of dark streets as they bobbed and bounced in search of treasure. The pirates, witches, dogs, and princesses wove tirelessly through the streets, up and down the steps of brightly lit houses. As they neared the end of their ritual hike, their homemade costumes told the story of being happy but worn out. Moms were urging, "This is the last stop," with bags and containers examined for inspection and comparison of their booty. But there is one more stop that a neighbor boy announced earlier to his friends: "My dad and my mom and I are having a haunted house a few blocks away in Dad's old house."

At the end of the street a gathering of night crawlers appeared, surrounding what looked like an old neglected two-story duplex with its top-floor windows boarded up, and below them flashing lights pierced the night giving the structure a creepy look. Upon our approach, all eyes were locked on a family of three: a tall thin cackling witch mother, a small dark-haired boy darting here and there with his impish grin, and a father with a knotted blood-soaked band crowning his head above a blood-streaked face. A gleaming steel axe blade in his right hand caught the light. The pirates, the witch, and the spotted dog stepped up to fill the space along the fence of people that bordered the front yard of the old building—now a stage for this trio.

With tilted heads and wide eyes, these creatures stared at the scene before them. The man menacingly crept toward the crowd, hissing and sneering with every step. Slowly turning his head, he locked eyes with the small pirate who stiffened and stepped back as the man made his approach. Miles, with eyes almost brimming with tears, placed his hand on his belted sword and did all that he could not to run towards me, his mother, as he stood beside the other costumed pirates, ghouls, and monsters.

An older boy shouted from the crowd, "Hey, that's my old house. That's my old room upstairs. You have no right to do this to my house."

Meanwhile, the man continued his approach, getting closer still to my son who remained with his friends but shouted, "Get away from me." With assurances from me and others near him that this is Joshua's dad, the little pirate stepped back toward the crowd. The other children widened the circle, with gaping mouths and eyes fastened on the man. All the while the squealing boy darted in and out of the empty house. The cackling witch glared at us through hollow windows with flickering light that pierced the night. The crowd stood still as the man stopped, turning his head away from the pirate, and then towards the small witch beside him. Without hesitation the little pirate stepped up, drew his tiny sword, and rushed the man. "Get away from my sister. Leave her alone or I'll kill you," he said. His voice did not waver. Pointing his sword, Miles swung wildly as he sprang toward the man. And then on bended knee, the man dropped his axe and gently spoke, "Miles, I'm Joshua's dad." But Miles did not hear him. Realizing the little pirate's fear, Joshua's dad removed his headband and wiped his face. The mother witch removed her hat. No longer frightened, the neighborhood children climbed through the windows of the empty house, with the impish boy leading the way. The angry boy, who had had many happy times there, turned back to shout once more, "You have no right to turn my house into a haunted sideshow."

With curtains drawn, lights dimmed, candies snuffed, and footsteps more measured than hours before the little pirate, the witch, and their friends and other creatures of the night, began their treks home. Miles quietly walked beside Lilly, with an occasional grumble that the man had better not come near his sister. Mr. Sadler had better be careful around him.

On a sunny afternoon some days later, Miles and Lilly spotted "the man" in our neighborhood park. Joshua had momentarily run back home, so his dad was alone. Mr. Sadler stopped to speak to the three of us. Miles stared at him directly in the face, pulled Lilly away, and stepped back himself. He repeated his warning, "You had better not bother my sister again." Mr. Sadler gently told him not to worry, that no one would hurt Lilly as long as her brother was nearby.

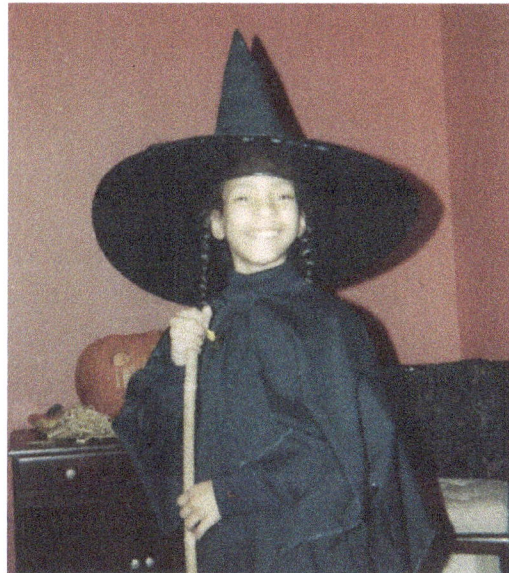

The Good Witch Lilly, Halloween 1990.

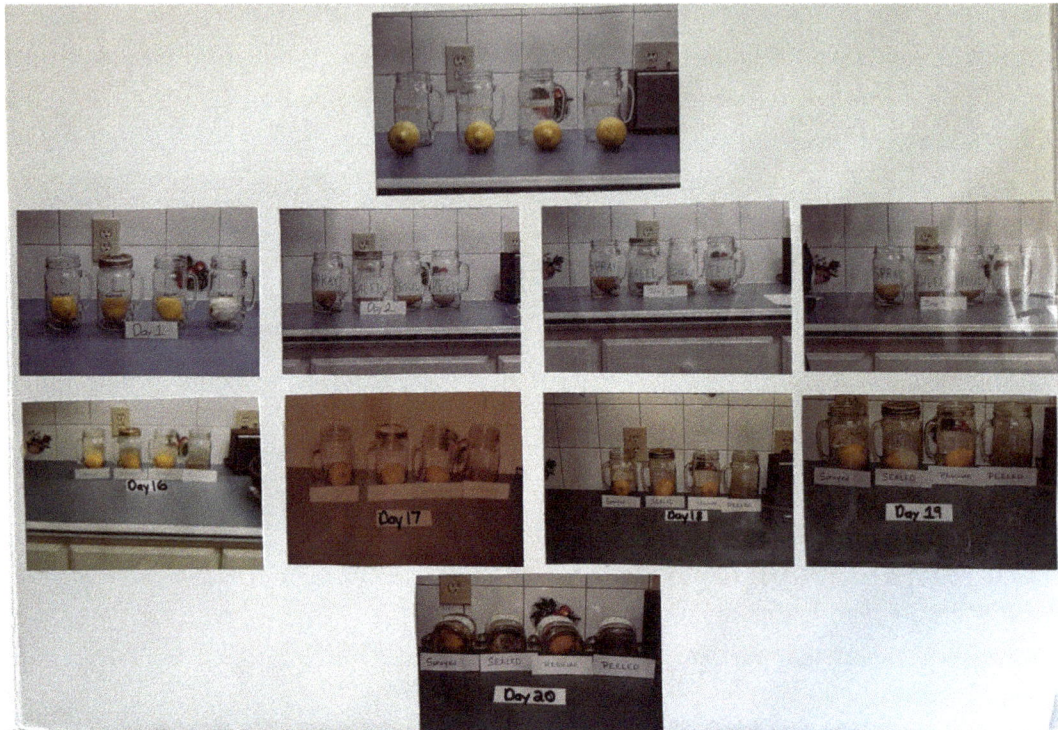

Lilly's Science Project.

The Trophy

Springtime in our household evokes memories of my children's annual school science projects. Third grade was one of those special times.

My eight-year-old son, Miles, was fascinated with electricity. Connecting electrical circuits to illuminate a light bulb put a gleam in his eye. Miles was a hands-on kind of kid—a tinkerer at heart. He would rather take something apart and put it back together, and leave the reasons why it worked up to someone else like his twin sister.

Lilly, anxious to start her science project, chose an obscure topic that interested her: the "preservation of lemons." She liked nothing more than sucking on a fresh slice of lemon after drinking a cold glass of Southern sweet tea. Her topic came from a science text some thirty years old, and its bibliography was far beyond the reach of our local public library, much less her school's small collection. Like a true scientist, Lilly read what little she could find, interviewed experts, and took many photographs of her experiment. Each day after school she rushed through our back door and headed straight to the kitchen counter where she painstakingly examined her lemons and charted her observations. Her efforts won her third place in the school's science fair, and made her eligible for the system-wide competition.

It was an unusually warm April day when Lilly, Miles, and I scrambled into the old blue van and quickly slid out of our narrow drive on our way to attend the big fair downtown. When we reached our destination—a huge old high school building in the center of Montgomery—we made our way through the long maze of exhibits that were carefully displayed in the school cafeteria. Along the way, Lilly and Miles spotted a number of their friends, also accompanied by their parents. As the crowd gathered, we meandered toward the large auditorium where the winners would be announced. Miles sat next to me while Lilly joined an enthusiastic group of her school chums.

As the auditorium filled with anxious children and their parents, a quiet hush fell over the room. The judges began their pronouncements. One by one as their names were called excited children bounced up and down from their seats, applauding themselves and their friends. Parents shared their pride. Then came the announcement: "Lilly Thompson, third grade, Forest Avenue School, honorable mention for physical science." It took Lilly

some time to make her way down what must have seemed like a mile-long aisle to accept her trophy. Miles and I could hardly contain ourselves—smiling and applauding her. Greeted by her cheering friends, Lilly rushed back to her seat—her face beaming with pride. Miles shouted out, "Let me see your trophy, Lilly." But she did not hear him.

Our trip home included the usual backseat banter. Who would hold the trophy? Lilly, wanting to savor the proof of her efforts, argued with her brother for what was rightfully hers.

When we arrived home, Lilly quietly slid upstairs to her room and placed her award among her other treasures—a dusty purple flower from her favorite babysitter, a homemade lamp from her aunt, and a small pink heart-shaped box she had made two summers ago. Later, Miles bounded up to her room where he immediately spotted the trophy. Despite Lilly's objections, he grabbed it from her dresser, getting his first real chance to examine it.

When I entered the room Miles's wide-eyed gaze was fixed on the object he held in his hand. He looked at Lilly and said, "Lilly, you won the first trophy in this house. May I take it to school tomorrow? I want to show it to my teacher."

I chimed in that she might want to show it to her teacher first. But Lilly reluctantly gave her consent.

The following morning, I accompanied Miles to his classroom where his teacher greeted him at the door. Immediately, he thrust the trophy into her hands while making his proclamation: "My sister, Lilly, won this at the science fair. She won the first

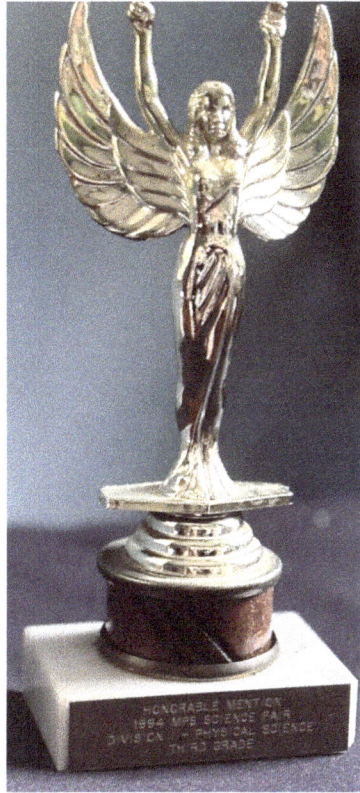

Lilly's trophy.

trophy in our house." Mrs. Turner gazed at him with a warm smile, and glanced up at me. Miles repeated the news to his classmates and proudly showed off the award.

On Sunday morning as we headed for church, I noticed that Miles again had taken the trophy from his sister's room. But this time there was only a slight protest from Lilly. During the morning announcements, Miles rose from his seat with Lilly's trophy held high, proclaiming that she had won it in the local science fair. Lilly was asked to stand and was given a healthy round of applause. In our hearts we applauded Miles too.

The Speech

One fall evening Lilly came home and announced that she was running for mayor of her fifth-grade class. She would make signs and give a speech at the end of the week. I was a bit surprised. Ordinarily, Lilly was rather quiet and reserved. She did not like to be the center of attention anywhere except at home where she expressed herself freely. For it was Lilly who called our family meetings and kept us all on task—creating art projects, preparing something special to eat, or playing school with her twin brother and their neighborhood friends. Lilly took charge. Family activities were her favorite. She liked nothing more than family dinners—just the day-to-day meals—when she expressed her ideas and told us about her day. Quite often, she and I were left at the table after her father and Miles had eaten and left. Lilly was busy talking, while the rest of us were eating and plotting who would get the leftovers from her plate.

Lilly's eyes—so lively and expressive—were dark brown deep pools that danced in the light. Though average height for a ten-year-old, she was quite thin. She ate mostly fruits and vegetables, even for snacks. Miles was about the same height but nearly twice her size.

After clearing the dinner dishes, Lilly and I made campaign signs and badges for her supporters. She coached me every step of the way. Her slogan—"honest and simple"—spoke for itself. "Vote for Lilly Thompson, a wise choice." When I asked why she wanted to be mayor and about her plans for the class, I immediately recalled how she had campaigned the summer before for more money for public schools. Marching from door-to-door with signs, she made sure we covered our street. We wore T-shirts bearing Lilly's views—"Help My School. We Support the New School Tax"—as she debated with some of her friends. But I did not know if Lilly had weighed the possibility of not winning her run for class mayor.

The morning sun bathed our kitchen as Lilly arose on campaign day. Dressed in an orange shorts set with tiny yellow flowers, she gathered her neatly stacked badges and signs from the kitchen table. When we arrived at her classroom I realized that I had not heard her speech. I lingered just long enough to feel that she was all right. She did not look back as I said goodbye, but continued to prepare for the day.

I returned to the school later that morning and took my place among a handful of other fifth-grade parents ready

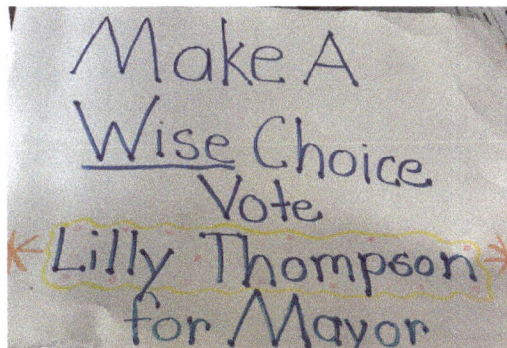

with cameras and seated on the edge of our chairs. I smiled and nodded towards Lilly seated on the stage with the other contenders. Her campaign banners, not nearly as elaborate as some others, were unmistakable to me. They were red and white and blue and white, with tiny dots at the end of each letter—seemingly a new fad in little girls' writing.

Lilly was the third or fourth candidate speaking that morning. The children clapped heartily after each speech. As her tiny figure glided towards the podium, I prayed that she would get the same reception. With erect posture, and eyes fixed on the audience, she spoke every word clearly.

It was obvious that she had written her own speech. She made no big promises—only those that she could keep—requesting a wider variety of Friday snacks and maintaining a cleaner classroom. I particularly remember her last promise—"I will try to be fair." I could have frozen that moment, for I was caught up in Lilly's simple display of courage and conviction.

And in an instant she was back in her seat adding another pair of swinging legs to the row of other mayoral contestants. Her face held a smile that was at once nervous, relieved, and responsive to the applause of her friends. I smiled at her and at the comments made by the parents about my daughter's candidacy and her speech. Other speeches followed Lilly's—some sounding very adult. But Lilly's was all her own.

With speeches now behind them, the children fell in line to return to their classrooms to vote. Although I could not get close enough to hug Lilly, I smiled at her for a job well done. For now she reserved that kind of display out of the sight of her friends. Regardless of the outcome, Lilly had come out a winner.

Exiting the school parking lot, I wondered how she felt. I wanted her to win the election because she had worked so solidly. When I picked up Miles at school that afternoon, he asked, "Did she win?" I told him he would be proud of his sister. For important issues, Miles was her biggest cheerleader.

That afternoon when Miles and I arrived at Forest Avenue, Lilly was standing outside with the others. I studied her face. Relieving her of her heavy backpack, my arm extended around her shoulder when she took the lead. In a tearful voice she said she'd lost the election. Miles immediately chimed in, "But Lilly, you were supposed to win."

Lilly did not dwell on the subject. She said she had a job to do. Lilly and some of the other mayoral contestants had won city council seats, and she had to get busy with her new job.

High Ropes Adventure

On a cool damp morning Forest Avenue's fifth grade students and their parents boarded the "Big Reds" parked just outside the school's side entrance. Once seated, Lilly, Miles, and I settled back to enjoy the ride with our respective partners—all headed for Camp Cosby, nestled in the Appalachian foothills of Alabama, for the annual fifth-grade retreat.

At the day's end, the teachers gladly passed the torch of responsibility for their students to chaperoning parents as they retreated to their more comfortable quarters. They left us clambering to the top bunks and the flickering flashlights of chatty little girls and boys too excited with each other's company to settle down to sleep.

The next morning was also cool and overcast as our group—Lilly and Miles among them—snaked through the woods to a clearing in the midst of tall Alabama pines. And there they were—the much-talked-about ropes course (talked about among parents primarily, and a particular dilemma for me) some sixty feet above our heads.

The ropes course cost an additional fee for any child wanting to tackle them. I paid for both children knowing that Miles would consider it an adventure and Lilly would have the option to choose. Her place was often beside me cheering for Miles and her dad as they relished the "wild rides" at the annual state fair.

As we approached the clearing, a small

group of maverick boys—with Miles among them—shot ahead to tackle their next adventure. They had geared up with protective harnesses and helmets as soon as we arrived. I spotted Miles as he was about to ascend the ropes far beyond my reach, far beyond my control, somewhere near the tops of those pines I once thought were so stately. As he scampered up the ladder he approached each section (which grew in difficulty) with the same fervor as he had the first. There was no uncertainty in his step. The last lap, the zip line, was a piece of cake for him to savor at the end. Before I realized it, he was on the ground laughing and talking with his friends, awaiting a second turn.

Meanwhile parents and teachers suited up the remaining line of girls. When Lilly's turn came, we searched for the smallest harness. She was clearly the smallest in her class. Nevertheless, she pulled on her gear, ready to make the climb with the others.

The children scampered up the ladder with Lilly chattering and joining her school chums. My eyes were glued on her tiny frame. The first part was quickly finished, and now the second—a bit more challenging—slowed this line of little girls until they reached the log, a single piece of rounded wood bridging the two most difficult parts of the course. When Lilly came to an abrupt halt so did my heart.

When the more daring girls reached the log, they seemed surprised. The choice was theirs, to cross the narrow bridge or fall off the log, abandoning the rest of the course. Many of these girls screeched with laughter as they enjoyed their brief suspension. I knew that Lilly would not. But I pulled back—a difficult task for me. The choice was hers.

I initially looked away, not wanting Lilly to have me choose for her. But honestly, the urge was tempting. She was sensitive to what my husband called my over-protectiveness. Many times I saw her pull back from her friends whenever we were together. However, lately I had seen such strides in her independence and self-confidence that I dared not interfere. I fought hard with my instinct to let her choose her own course. With each passing moment, I realized that the choice was as difficult for her as it was for me.

As Lilly began her careful journey across the bridge she took a step backward—no rails or ropes to hold on to, only the belt of the safety harness. Meg tilted sideways and fell off the log, dangling by the hook until she was unharnessed. Some others followed suit. A few decided to stay the course. Lilly was among them.

She continued. Reaching the next platform, she turned around and froze. Shouts from below encouraged her to keep on. We

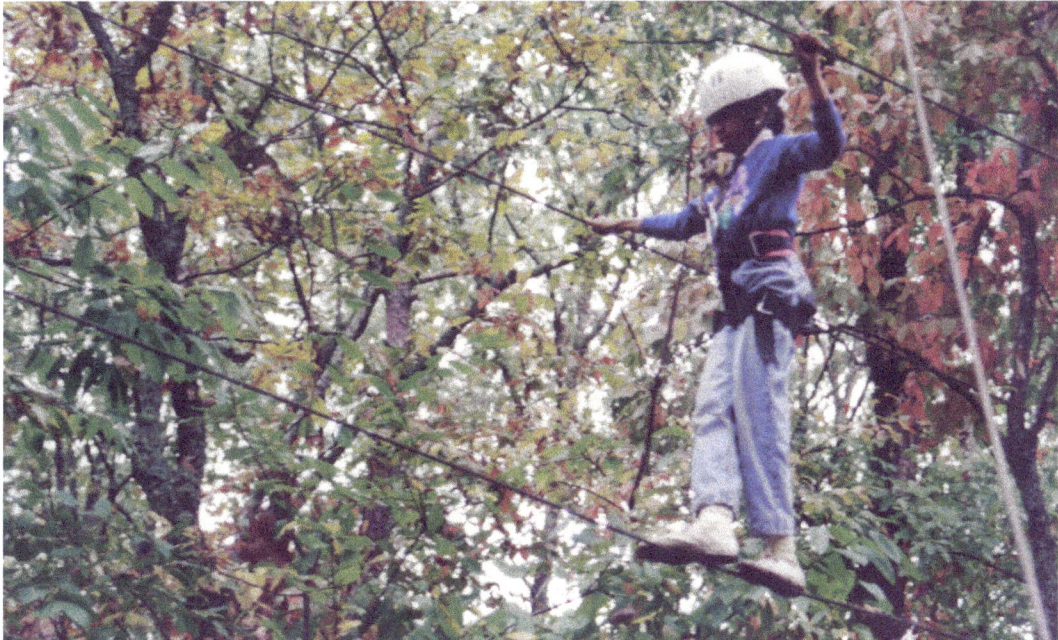

One foot before the other, Lilly made her way. My heart was in my throat.

were all focused on her hesitant ascent, one foot before the other. The line of those waiting suddenly fell silent for all eyes were on Lilly. Her teacher stood directly under her urging her to take one more step. I stood away to get a wider view, holding back for a while before joining in the cheers. I heard my heart pounding and grasped at my collar. One step forward, one step back—Lilly's tiny body was quivering amid the shouts of encouragement. She would not choose to fall down. I looked to her teacher and then back to Lilly—*couldn't someone get her down?* She had reached the point of no return as her classmates were piling up behind her. Shouts from her friends on the ground gradually turned into impatience. Lilly was concentrating with such intensity that I felt her apprehension.

My fear mounted. *Couldn't someone get her down? Enough was enough.* I realized that she had made her decision and no one could get her down now. Her tiny frame came to the last course where she met with the instructor on a lofty pole. The line of children on the log was slowly beginning to move. And the shouts from below began again. "Come on, Lilly, this is the fun part." After continuous urging from her peers and the instructor poised at the top, Lilly began her descent down the zip line in an eerie silence. I snapped a blurry picture for her to keep as one of the bravest things she's ever done. I felt for sure that she thought this was the end.

When she hit the ground, her knees must have buckled, for we both stood frozen. After she caught her breath, I embraced her so tightly. I could not let her go. In my heart I was apologizing to her for allowing this to happen. But Lilly stood up, brushed herself off, and took off with her friends, bragging how she made it to the end. Her peers cheered and must have talked about the feat for the rest of the night. Afterwards, one parent, Gladys Gillis, who had sworn she would never try to make it across, climbed onto the course and completed it. She said Lilly had given her the courage to try.

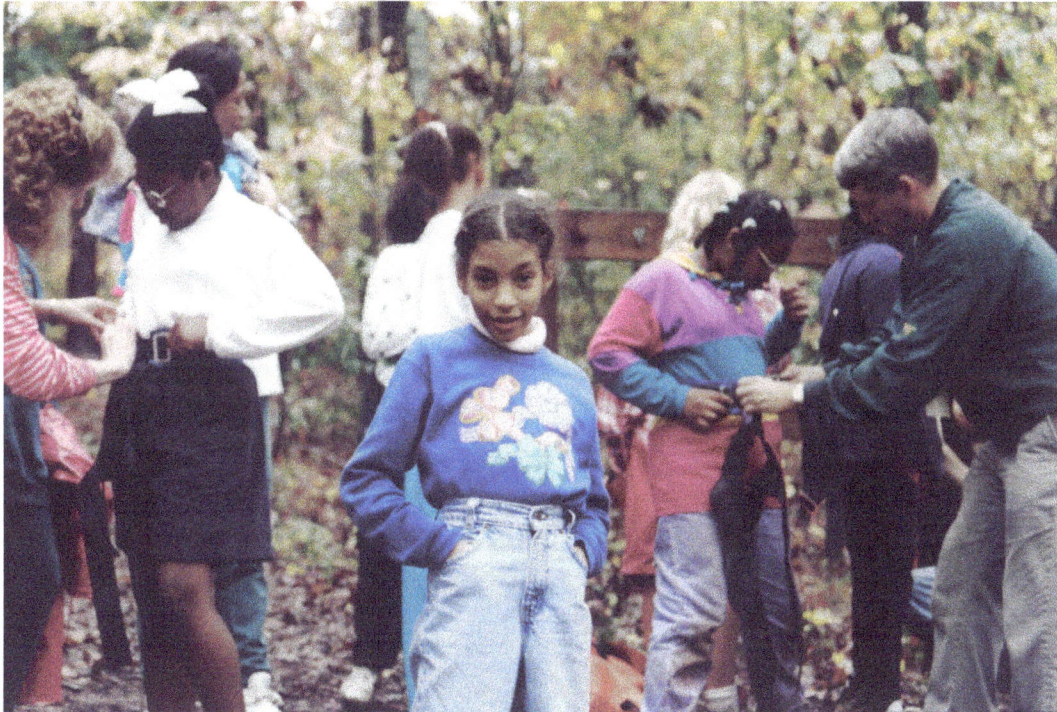

Lilly had to choose whether to do the ropes course. And she made the choice.

History of the Lilly Thompson Garden and Outdoor Classroom

After an art competition sponsored by the Clean City Commission, a Forest Avenue School student who entered the contest started a club among her friends. Five or six rising third graders met that summer in one another's homes to determine their mission and elect officers. They dubbed themselves the "Save the Earth Club."

Dana Siegelman, who had the idea, was elected president. My daughter, Lilly Thompson, was vice president, and her twin brother, Miles, was treasurer. With recycling their main focus, the children collected newspapers and aluminum cans from family and friends, gathered trash from the neighborhood park, set up a bank account, and planned field trips that helped them understand the purpose and methods of recycling.

In the summer heat, the group toured a local landfill, visited two recycling plants, and subscribed to an environmental magazine through the Waste Management Recycling Company. The newspapers and cans they collected were submitted to the company for cash that was deposited into the club's bank account.

"Miss Lilly's School" was also in session at our house. Several neighborhood children gathered in our front room for math, reading, and field trips to the neighborhood park to pick up trash and collect acorns, rocks, and bird feathers. The ditch that runs through this park was a gold mine of interesting creatures—tadpoles and turtles—to be brought home and examined. Wildflowers along the roadside were just waiting to be picked. Homemade bird food, concocted from

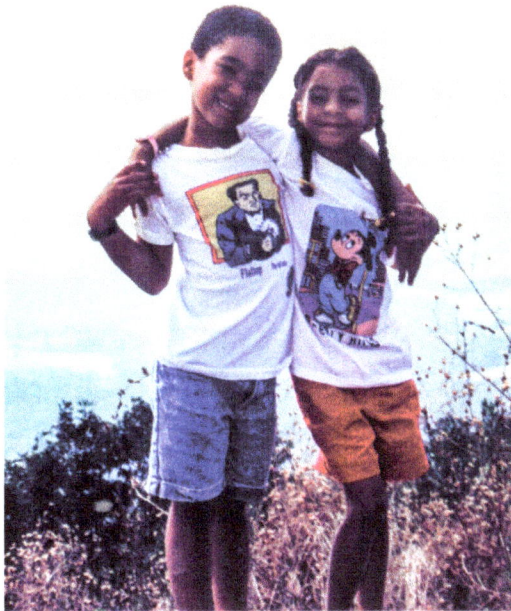

Miles and Lilly on one of our road trips.

recipes in our kitchen, was hung on tree branches. The children constructed floating boats of leaves and sticks that eventually made their way to our back porch. Miles readily obliged his sister, pulling the girls all through the park in his and Lilly's red wagon to enhance their collections.

During car trips from Montgomery to the Alabama coast, Lilly insisted on stopping to gather the beautiful red clover that lined the highway. Our stops at welcome centers were another collection point. Paper and wild flowers filled the back seat below her feet. In the early spring, our backyard was brightened with tiny wild white lilies that we dared not mow. With the help of Lilly's science teacher, Sherry White, cicadas, butterflies, beetles, moths, and grasshoppers were found and mounted. With a backyard full of trees that drew all sorts of birds, Lilly requested a children's field guide to consult for bird identification. Scattered feathers were saved for yet another collection and sometimes incorporated into homemade costumes. Nature was Lilly's playground and her school.

With summer ended, the Save the Earth Club third-graders took their recycling project to Forest Avenue principal Maggie Stringer. Before we knew it, the collection of recycled materials had gone school-wide. Under her leadership, with teachers, and parents on board, classes competed to raise the most money from their recyclables. Monthly ice cream and pizza parties were held for the winners. The school buzzed with activity. With homemade signs, club members hawked recyclables at the curb as other students spilled out of their cars for morning classes. Parents placed recycling containers outside each classroom and collected the contents each Friday.

The recycling campaign was now a part of the school culture, and it had spread to Dannelly Elementary School where Miles was enrolled. With their recycling earnings, Dannelly's third graders purchased bedding plants for a lovely flower garden to beautify a barren area of their school's front lawn.

The following year, under the leadership of Susan Seagraves, Dannelly School won a large grant from the Junior League that enabled the construction of an environmental center complete with various natural habitats, a water feature, and a classroom with lab equipment specifically designed to study environmental science. Parents and students worked hard to prepare the area.

Meanwhile, Forest Avenue students continued their recycling campaign. In the fall of 1995 the new fifth graders, of which Lilly was one, headed north to Camp Cosby for two days of bonding, nature study, and Alabama history—a fifth-grade tradition established by School Principal Mrs. Maggie Stringer. This was the last outing that Lilly had with her classmates.

Lilly's memorial service was held at Forest Avenue, when the fifth grade announced that the proceeds from the school's recycling efforts would be used to establish a garden in her name. The "Lilly Pad" was a gift that the Class of 1997 left to their school in the name of their late

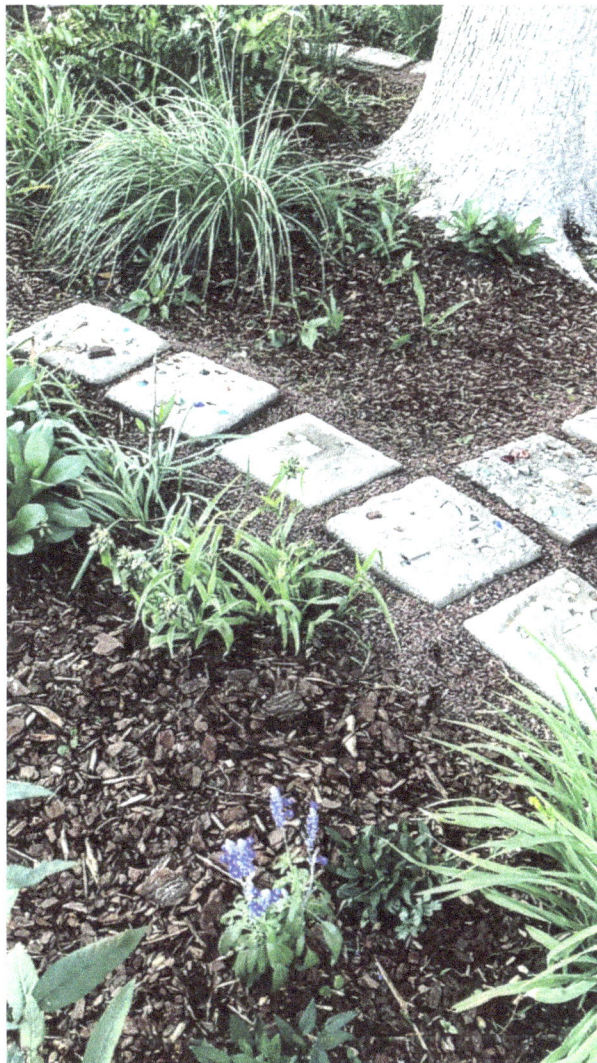

classmate. The ribbon-cutting service was held on May 16, 1997.

Under the leadership of Principal Maggie Stringer, the school used the garden as an outdoor classroom. The children of Forest Avenue School have studied plant life and wild birds, set up a sundial, made birdhouses from gourds, created stepping stones with beautiful colors, and grown vegetables. The garden creates many opportunities that incorporate every phase of the school's curriculum.

Our hope is that the tradition established through the collaborative efforts of many persons will continue, that the Lilly Pad will be a lasting place of learning for children while maintaining its natural beauty. Our family cannot think of a more fitting way to honor our Lilly.

Stepping stones were crafted by students and placed in the "outdoor classroom."

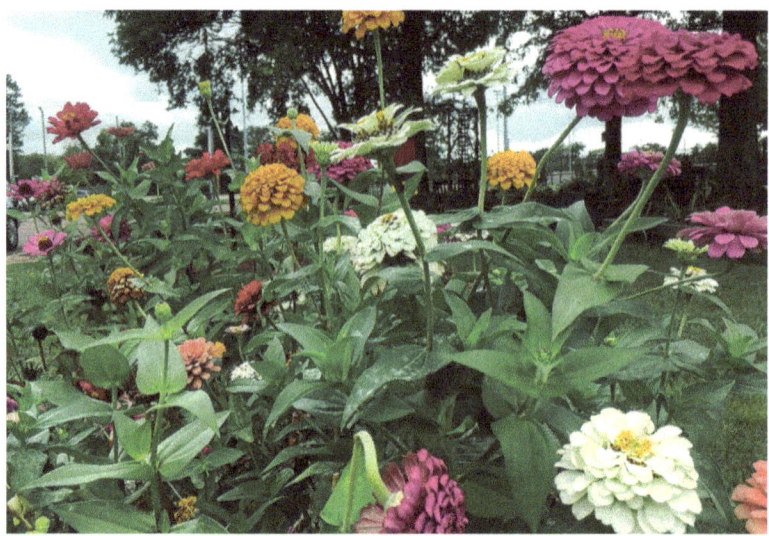

Scenes from Lilly's Garden, 1997 to Present. Bottom right, May 16, 1997, dedication ceremony held by her 6th grade graduating class.

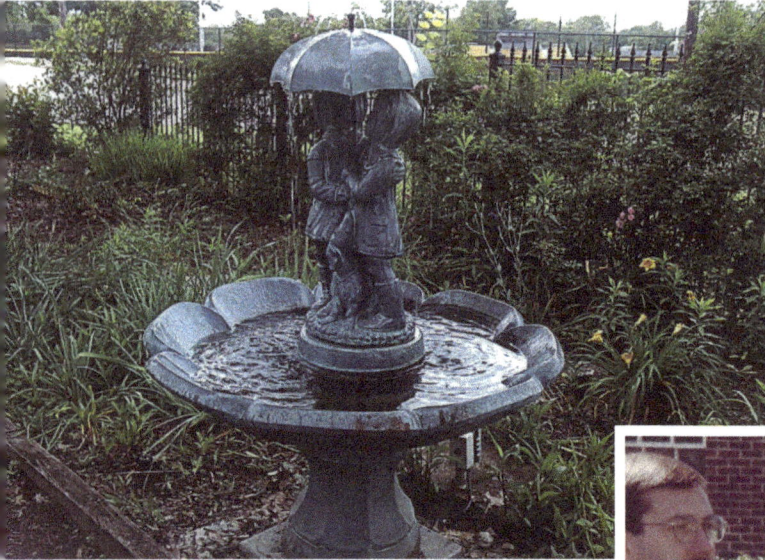

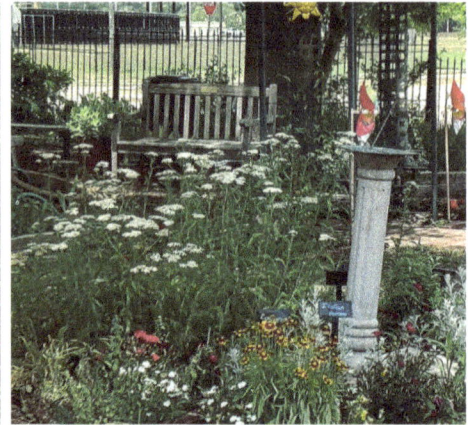

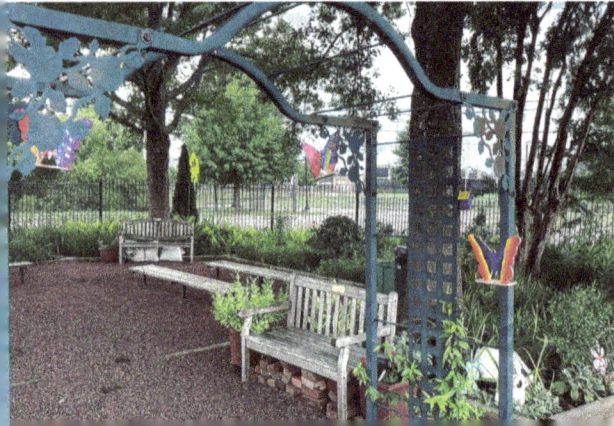

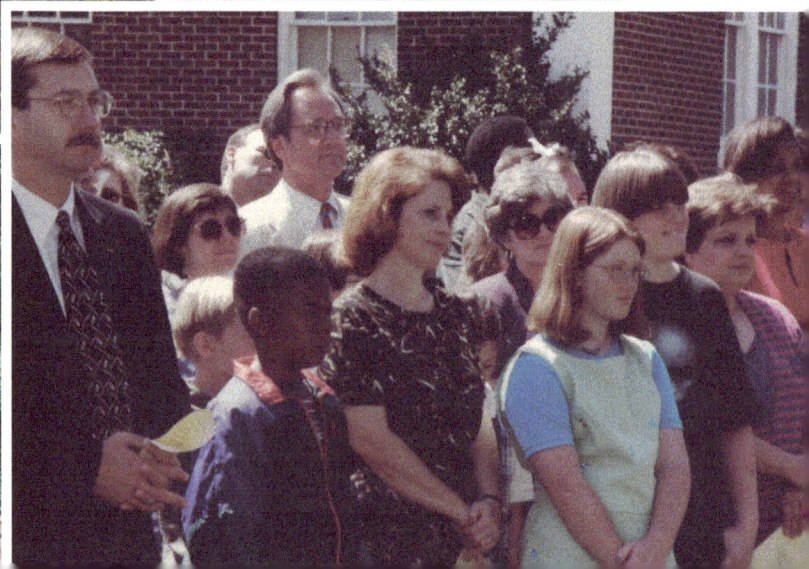

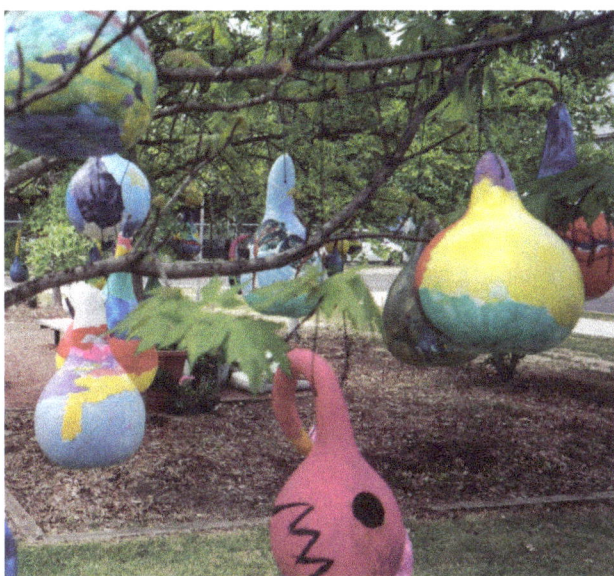

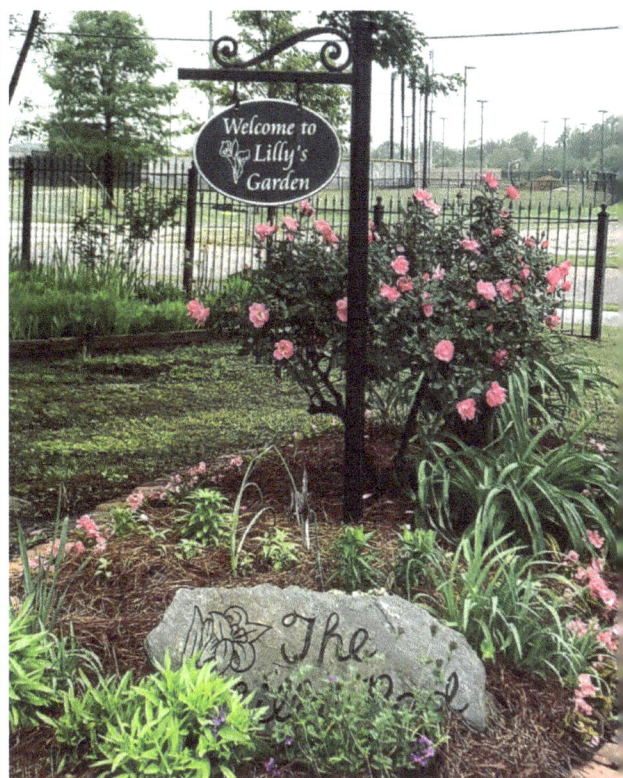

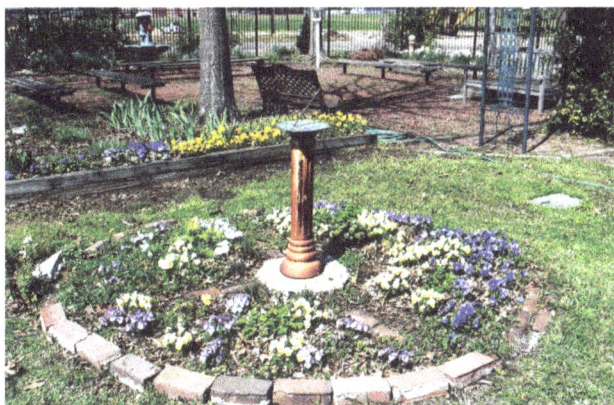

Clockwise from above: Entrance; 4th grade birdhouse project; the Maggie Stringer Sun Dial; and gourds painted by the 4th grade.

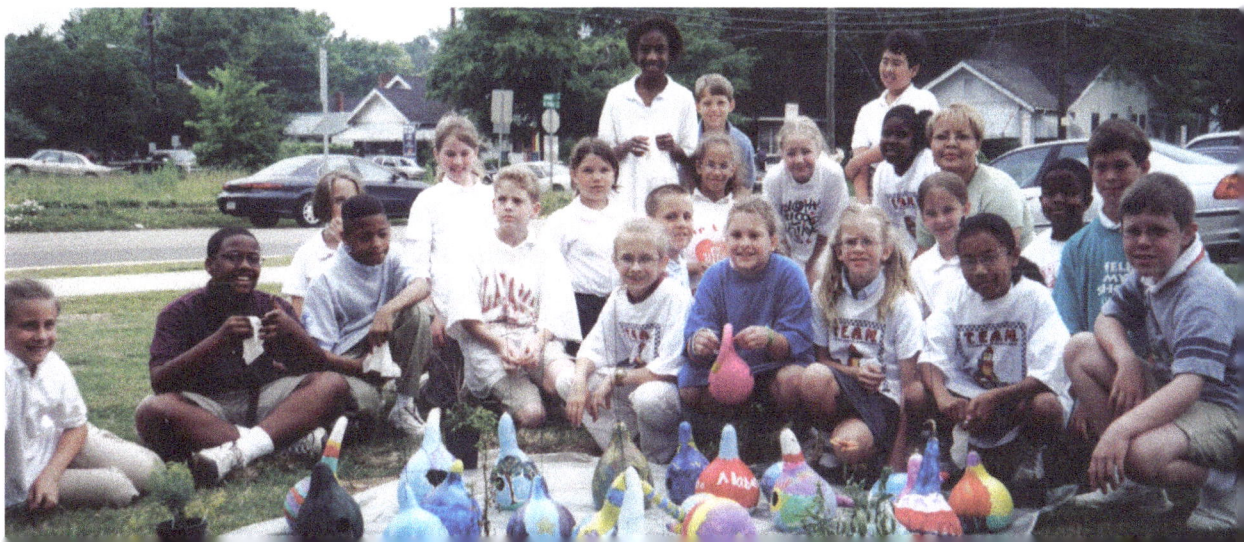

Acknowledgments

A huge thank-you to Mrs. Maggie Stringer, the now retired principal of Forest Avenue Acadcmic Magnet Elementary School, who listened to the needs and desires of her students when they suggested that their school begin a recycling program to help the environment and raise money for a school garden. Mrs. Stringer advocated for her students, bringing the teachers and parents on board to support this project. In addition, Mrs. Stringer sought the help of the Capital City Master Gardeners who, to this day, work voluntarily to beautify the garden and provide activities for the students. She has been a strong advocate for the garden for twenty-eight years. In 2025, the school and community celebrated Mrs. Stringer's ninetieth birthday in Lilly's Garden.

Thank you to the Siegelman family, who paved the way to complete the garden for school use. Lori Siegelman encouraged her daughter, Dana, to enter an art contest sponsored by the Clean City Commission for elementary schools to challenge their students by drawing pictures that represented ways to keep our city clean. Dana won that contest for her school and later obtained her mother's permission to form a club of third-grade classmates

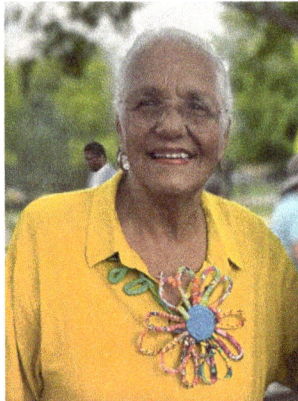

Mrs. Stringer.

that met throughout the summer, studied the environment, worked to keep it clean, and recycled newspaper and aluminum cans collected from their neighborhoods. The children dubbed their group the Save the Earth Club. They decided to put their money towards a school garden. Thank you to the members of the club for taking a small idea and creating a vision for something greater. And thank you to all graduating sixth-grade students of the Forest Avenue Class of 1997 for a dream come true for all the students at their school.

Thank you to Shirley Johnson, the now retired school counselor who found ways to engage the teachers to use the garden as an outdoor classroom and expand their curricula with hands-on experiences for all six grades at the school. Mrs. Johnson was the true liaison between the Master Gardeners and the teachers. Her leadership helped engage school parents and clubs such as Girl Scouts and Jack and Jill of America to volunteer not only in garden upkeep but also in planned activities. She found effective ways to raise money for Lilly's Garden. Although she has long since retired from the school, she still offers valuable support.

Thank you to Margaret Barber, an artist and parent volunteer who used her skills as a potter and experience working with young children to chair our garden committee for a year. Margaret's work was vital not only in garden upkeep but also in planning activities that were both educational and fun.

Thank you to Janet Woods, president of the school's PTA, who recruited parent volunteers of which she was a part. She helped plan and execute activities to promote garden use and raise money as well. Janet encouraged me to seek a publisher who could advise me about sharing my stories.

Thank you to the many volunteers from Capital City Master Gardeners (CCMGA) who spent time working and planning activities, donating funds for school projects, and maintaining the garden, including repairing the hardscape, installing new benches, and maintaining our Little Free Library. Because of the hard work of this group, Lilly's Garden was the recipient of the Alabama Master Gardener Association's "Search for Excellence Award" in 2014. A lengthy and time-consuming proposal completed by former member Brenda Coleman helped us receive the award.

A special thank-you to Paul Furr who hybridized *Lilly's Smile* in 2012. This beautiful hardy daylily is the blooming star of Lilly's Garden. In May 2025, Jane Martin donated a beautiful daylily, *Miles's Smile (Sargent)*, that is planted near *Lilly's Smile*. The two appear as alike as the brother and sister they represent.

A huge thank-you to the chairs and co-chairs of Lilly's Garden—Suzanne Reeves, Janice Jackson, and Billie Crawford. Billie thinks nothing is impossible. All of these volunteers are so encouraging.

Thank you to Forest Avenue teachers and parents, and Huntingdon College students (the latter led by Chris Clark) who donated time and plants to the garden. Many thanks to Paula Johnson, who maintained the garden for two years prior to its official adoption by CCMGA.

Special thank-yous to many personal friends, too numerous to mention here, who celebrated the good times as well as stood by us in difficult times. Thank you to Aquila, who after leading Forest Avenue students in a school-wide quilting project, taught Lilly to crochet and quilt—two of her favorite hobbies. And a special thank-you to Teresa and Lynn who replanted the school yard in front of Dannelly School (where Miles attended) when our family lost Lilly.

Thank you to Candice and her son, Dylan McBroom, for blessing Miles's life with a godson, and my life with a grand-godson since he was six months old. Dylan is truly a bright light in my life.

Thank you to Miles's friends who surrounded us with support and caring upon his passing.

Thank you to our church family who

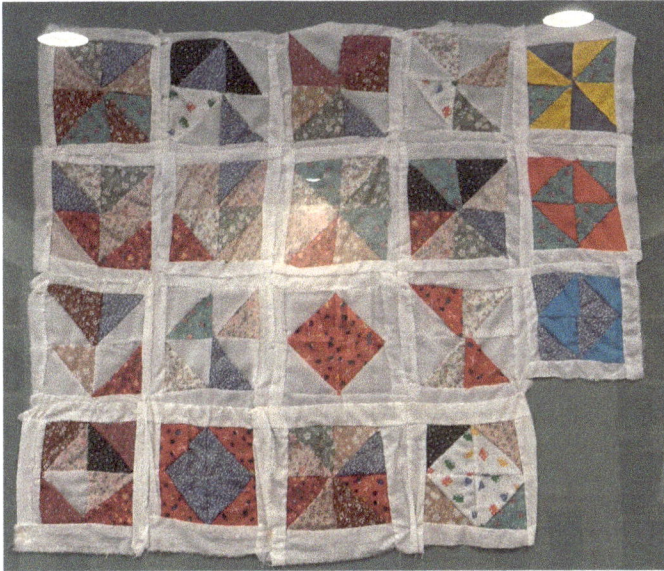

Lilly's unfinished quilt, made in the fourth grade with the help of "Aunt Aquila."

I can never forget Myron's law clerks and our law clerk family, along with Lillian Thomas. You have always been loving and supportive of Myron, our children, and me, and you continue to be so through the years.

Thank you to Nancy Anderson, retired AUM professor, who unknowingly helped me learn to channel my grief through writing stories about my children.

This book would not have been published without the guidance, assistance, and encouragement of friends Suzanne La Rosa and Randall Williams. I cannot thank them enough for their perseverance through all of our unexpected challenges.

supported us through challenges in our lives we could never have imagined and helped me give my children a moral compass to live by. And a special thank-you to my children's grandparents, who were so excited when they were born, and to other extended family members who always stand with us.

And last but by no means least, Trey Granger, who no matter what will always get the work done, and done well, in his very kind way. Thank you so much, Trey.

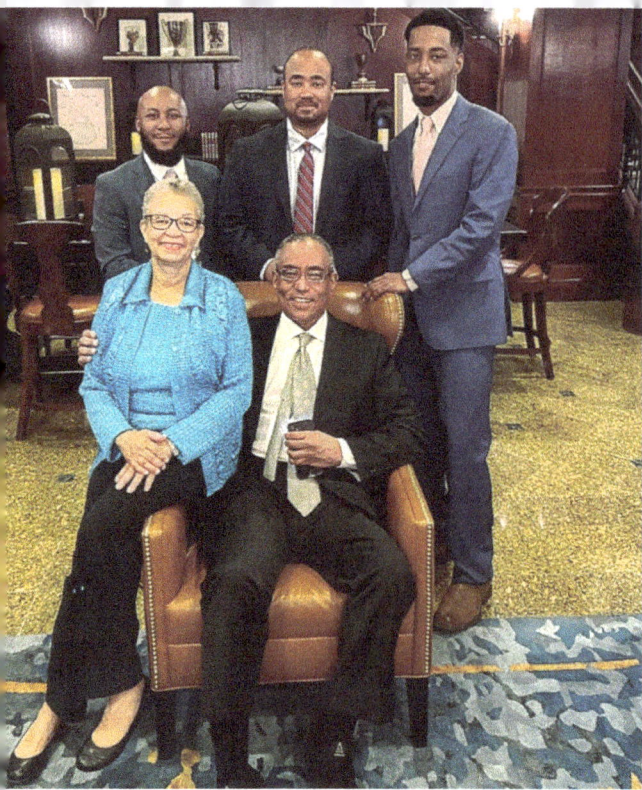
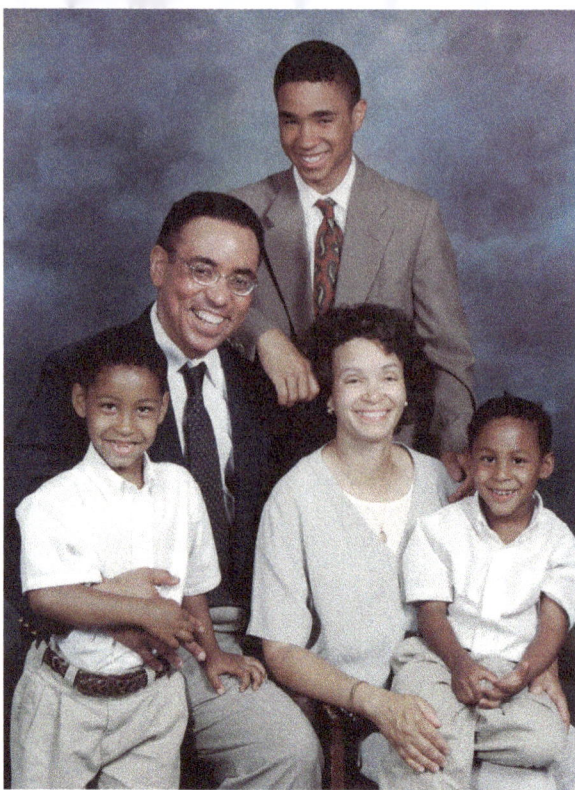

Above right: Our new family in 1999 on the baptism of our two youngest children, Jason and Jaylan Thompson. Above left and below: We celebrated in 2022 as Myron received an honorary doctorate from his alma mater, Yale College.

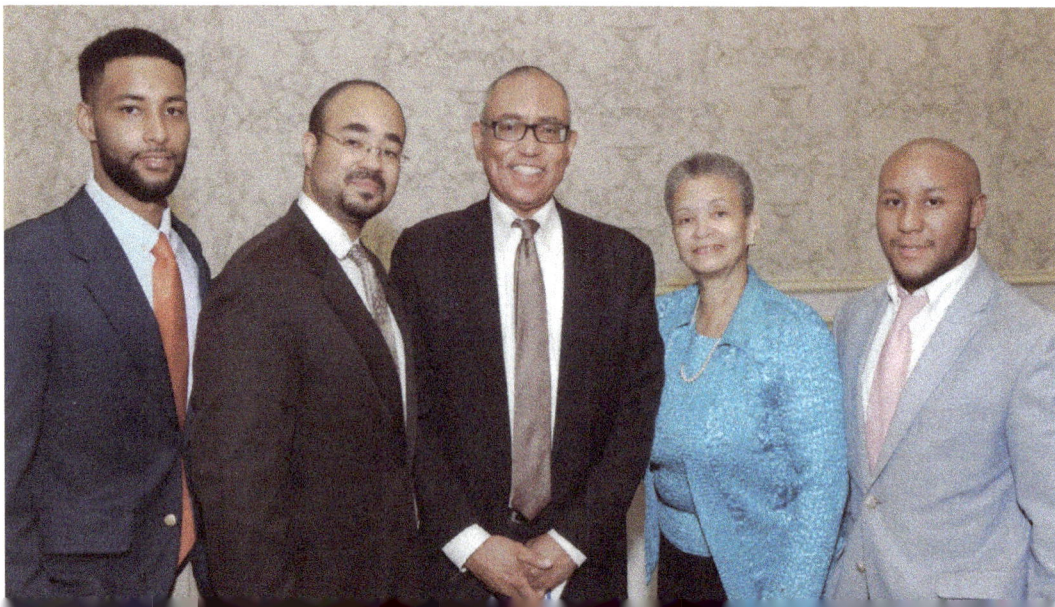

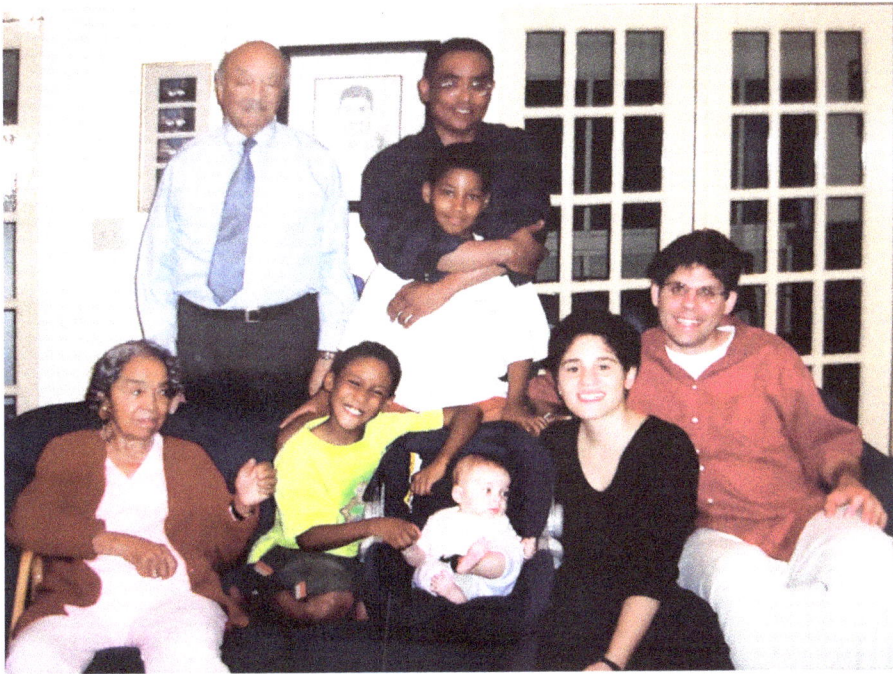

Top, fun with the clerks and grandparents.

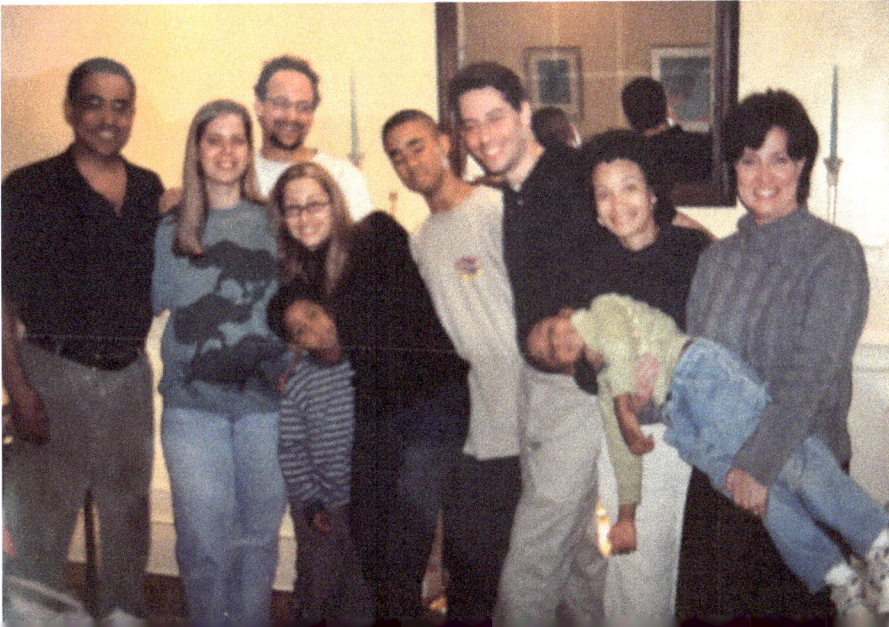

Bottom, more members of our "law clerk family" over the years.

www.ingramcontent.com/pod-product-compliance
Lightning Source LLC
Chambersburg PA
CBHW041604260326
41914CB00012B/1385